Perfect Match

A Kidney Transplant Reveals
the Ultimate Second Chance

Janet Hermans

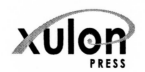

Dedicated to Erik,
and
kidney donors everywhere.

Special thanks to
doctors, nurses,
researchers and
other medical professionals
who work to improve
patients' lives,
and also to organizations
like the National
Transplant Assistance Fund
that help make
second chances possible.

Acknowledgements

*P*erfect Match was finally published because of the urging of my mother, Chris Frey. Thank you, Mom, for your encouragement, persistence and support.

My documents were corrected numerous times by my friend and husband, Hans. Thank you, Buddy, for your honesty, patience and good sense.

Perfect Match was edited by various people who corrected grammar and/or provided constructive criticism. Thank you Mom and Dad Hermans, Mom and Dad Frey, Jay and Leslie Miller, Debbie Salas,

Tom Carson, Monica Beck, Bob Palumbo, Doreen Yeremian and Lydia Krieger.

Some friends in an Alpha course were great sounding boards as I developed the parallels found in this book. Thank you Donna Dolbashian, Christie Dingman and Doreen Yeremian.

Table of Contents

Introduction xi

Chapter 1a: Erik's Choice 15
Chapter 1b: Jesus' Choice 21

Chapter 2a: Erik Paves the Way 29
Chapter 2b: Jesus Paves the Way 33

Chapter 3a: Erik's Suffering 41
Chapter 3b: Jesus' Suffering 45

Chapter 4a: Hans' Transformation 51
Chapter 4b: Our Transformation 55

Chapter 5a: Erik's Recovery 63

Chapter 5b: Jesus' Resurrection.............................65

Chapter 6a: Adjusting to the Kidney.....................71

Chapter 6b: Living with the Spirit 75

Chapter 7a: Becoming Like Erik 83

Chapter 7b: Becoming Like Jesus...........................87

Chapter 8a: Perfect Match 93

Chapter 8b: Perfect Match 97

Endnote 105

Introduction

*P*erfect Match is written in parallel chapters to illustrate the love of Jesus and the transforming work of the Holy Spirit through the account of my husband's kidney transplant. I hope it offers encouragement and clarification to your life whether you are someone searching for God, a new believer or one who has walked with God for many years.

The details of my husband's medical record are not essential to this book. Many people suffer from kidney disease or other illnesses that destroy the kidneys. Hans got sick as a teenager and lived with reduced kidney function for 20 years. He is one of the fortunate ones who received a transplant.

Greater love
has no one than this,
that he lay down his life
for his friends.
John 15:13

Chapter 1a:
Erik's Choice

On Monday September 6, 1999, our family drove to the Hospital of the University of Pennsylvania in Philadelphia. Our children were amazed at the size of the facility. Evan, age four, loved the huge parking garage with all its car ramps. Leslie, six, enjoyed the long glass tunnel that bridged the street. Hansy, eight, liked the Italian hoagies in the big cafeteria.

We went through a maze of hallways, lobbies, elevators and escalators until we found the floor of the correct high-rise building to which my husband Hans and his brother Erik had been assigned. Their rooms were completely different. Hans, the kidney recipient, had a small, standard single across from the nurses' station. Erik, the kidney donor, was given a large corner suite with extra seating and a coffee table. The big windows gave it a more cheerful atmosphere than most hospital rooms.

Naturally, it was in Erik's suite that the extended family congregated. There were fifteen of us in and out of Erik's room over the next several days, and nearly all of us were there the first evening, giving it an intimate, party-like atmosphere.

Several family members were surprised to learn that Hans' kidney transplant was not like fixing a car; his kidneys would not be repaired, or removed and replaced. Instead, his existing kidneys would be left untouched, while Erik's kidney would be inserted under Hans' pelvic muscles!

With this information in mind, I quizzed Hansy: "How many kidneys does Daddy have?"

"Two," our oldest son answered hesitantly.

"That's right. How many kidneys does Uncle Erik have?"

"Two," he answered again.

"How many of Dad's kidneys work?" I continued.

"I don't know. I don't think they work, do they?"

"No, they don't. They barely work at all, so I guess the answer is zero. But how many of Uncle Erik's kidneys work?"

"Two?" he answered tentatively.

"Yes, we sure hope so! Now, it gets tricky. How many kidneys will Dad have tomorrow?"

Hansy didn't miss a beat. "Three!"

"So how many kidneys will Uncle Erik have tomorrow?"

"One!" he announced triumphantly.

Everyone was laughing at this cute arithmetic lesson. It seemed amusing at first, but I felt tension building in the room. Although Hans was feeling optimistic about receiving the solution to his illness, Erik was becoming increasingly anxious.

Of Hans' four younger brothers, Erik had been completely sure before his blood was even tested that he would be "it" — the one to donate. Sure enough, he'd tested as a perfect match. Now though, he was faced with the imminent reality of the handoff. "Uncle Erik will have one kidney tomorrow… one kidney… one…"

I imagined Erik hopping out of bed and making a run for it. He wasn't sick. He didn't owe us anything. He hadn't signed a contract or been paid to donate a kidney. The only thing he had been guaranteed was more pain and discomfort than Hans, because a kidney transplant is usually more difficult for the donor.

As I considered Erik's growing anxiety, I became uneasy because I realized Hans' health rested entirely with Erik's voluntary decision. Erik had no obligation to continue. Since no one was forcing him to donate, I wouldn't have blamed him if he'd lost his nerve and gone home. As much as Erik felt he was "it" — the one to donate, he still didn't *have* to. What would happen if he changed his mind and left? My mind clouded with worries. My husband's future quality of life hung precariously on Erik's choice....

I snapped out of my daydream and shot a glance across the room at Erik. He still looked nervous, but he wasn't going anywhere. I felt so grateful he was choosing to go ahead with the transplant. For the first time I really understood and appreciated the weight of the decision Erik had made in donating a kidney to Hans. Knowing that he had chosen to do this, not by force or obligation, made what he was about to do all the more incredible to me.

Chapter 1b:
Jesus' Choice

Over 2000 years ago Jesus gathered with his friends, not in a hospital room, but in a large upper room in Jerusalem to celebrate the Passover. All the preparations had been made. It was to be a joyous time of fellowship away from the crowds, but since Jesus knew he would die soon, it was also a solemn occasion. I imagine there was talking and joking as in Erik's room. We know from Luke's gospel the disciples' conversation digressed to arguing about who was the greatest.

Meanwhile, Jesus was about to face the hardest trial of his life. Here his friends were competing, completely missing the point. Prior to that evening, Jesus had told them that when he came to Jerusalem he would suffer and be put to death, but on the third day he would rise from the dead. The disciples didn't understand. They were not able to fathom that the same Jesus who healed the sick, performed miracles and was the Messiah, would suffer and die. Instead, they wanted and expected Jesus to overthrow their Roman oppressors.

Now in this upper room, Jesus spoke to his disciples again regarding his mission. Through the Passover meal, he explained that the bread and wine were his body and blood. He communicated the necessity to give himself: his body would be broken and his blood shed, and he would become the perfect Passover lamb.

I wonder, at any point during his ministry and especially now that the crucifixion was imminent, if Jesus ever considered leaving as I imagined Erik doing. Jesus could have. He knew he was "it" — the One to save the world, but no one was forcing him.

Shortly after the meal, Jesus took his disciples to the garden of Gethsemane. He chose three of them to be near him while he prayed. He was deeply troubled and totally overwhelmed, and he wanted them to keep watch while he prepared himself for the upcoming events. Jesus fell with his face to the ground praying, "Father, if it is possible, take this cup from me. Yet not as I will, but as you will."

Jesus was in anguish as he prayed because he had a choice regarding his sacrifice. Just as Erik made a freewill decision to donate a kidney, Jesus made a freewill decision to lay down his life.

When Jesus checked on his friends, they were asleep. He woke them saying, "Could you men not keep watch with me for one hour? Watch and pray so that you will not fall into temptation. The spirit is willing but the body is weak." (Matthew 26:40-41)

This rebuke was directed at his three sleepy friends, but on another level Jesus may have been experiencing this struggle himself. His divine spirit was willing, but his human flesh was screaming, "No!!"

He knew, because he was the Son of God, what lay ahead, and it was horrible. He already knew of his coming betrayal, knew his disciples would abandon him, knew Peter would deny him, knew he would be scourged, mocked, crucified and separated from God for the first time ever. And because Jesus was also fully human, he would feel the full spectrum of pain like any normal person. His humanity also gave him the free will to refuse it all. What an enormous temptation avoiding the cross must have been!

Jesus could have walked away from the cross as surely as Erik could have walked out of the hospital. But Jesus prayed three times in Gethsemane and submitted himself fully to God's will. It was an excruciatingly difficult decision.

It's humbling and amazing to consider that Jesus chose crucifixion to remedy sin. And realizing he was not forced, but gave his life willingly, warrants our love and gratitude.

The accounts of Jesus' last Passover supper and struggle in Gethsemane are found in Matthew 26, Mark 14 and Luke 22. Jesus' deity and humanity are discussed in John 1, Philippians 2, Colossians 1, Hebrews, and throughout the Scriptures.

Very rarely
will anyone die for a
righteous man, though for a
good man someone might
possibly dare to die. But God
demonstrates his own love for
us in this: while we were still
sinners, Christ died for us.
Romans 5:7-8

For it is by grace
you have been saved,
through faith – and this is not
from yourselves, it is the
gift of God – not by works,
so that no one can boast.
Ephesians 2:8-9

Chapter 2a:
Erik Paves the Way

The next day finally came, Tuesday September 7. To my relief, neither Erik nor Hans had left during the night. Both were jittery though: Hans, because of toxins running through his system due to failing kidneys, and Erik because of nervousness.

Their mother, Ann, was feeling most nervous of all. Two of her grown boys were having surgery on the same day. She was concerned about Erik because he'd had abdominal surgery as a toddler. Even 25 years later the long, thick scar was a strong visual reminder that his surgery and healing had been difficult. Did Erik have internal scarring that would interfere with today's surgery? Would his new wounds, internal and external, heal well?

Ann was also concerned about Hans. She felt so much was at stake because Hans had three young children and managed a growing company. The success of the surgery would affect not only Hans' life, but his family and employees as well.

In a kidney transplant, the donor does his part first, so Erik went into surgery before Hans. Ann gave this account: "Early in the morning, the hospital staff came to get Erik from his room, and he climbed on the gurney. As they wheeled him away, I stood at the end of the hall watching him disappear through the doors, separating me from him, and him from our support.

"Erik told me later that he was wheeled directly into the operating theatre, and the entire medical team was there in their green surgical scrubs, masks and caps, ready to "pounce" on him. Then there was a delay because of some problem with equipment or retesting of his blood. It was then it hit Erik the hardest, and he begged the doctors to put him under with the anesthesia. Although not *physically* painful, the anticipation of what lay ahead in that room surrounded by strangers was the worst and most nerve wrecking aspect of the entire ordeal."

The doctors planned to remove Erik's kidney using laparoscopic surgery. This method would spare him the removal of a rib and a huge incision from his belly button to his backbone. The surgeons succeeded, resulting in what brother Paul described later as a shark bite: seven half-inch cuts for inserting probes and tools, and one three-inch cut through which the kidney was removed.

Erik's choice to donate a kidney was the focus of the last chapter. Hans had a choice too: whether to accept the kidney or not. It was an easy decision because Hans understood his condition and the limitations of dialysis. He knew Erik's kidney gave hope for a new lease on life. Receiving Erik's kidney was clearly the way to go.

Still, it was a choice. At the point that Erik was in surgery, but before Hans was anesthetized, Hans could have backed out. He could have walked away, rejecting the kidney out of fear of having another surgery or needing general anesthesia and "going under."

But of course, Hans received the kidney as planned. Like Erik, he said goodbye to his mother and was wheeled into the operating room. The surgeon put Erik's kidney in Hans' pelvic cavity and hooked it up to filter Hans' blood. His own, low functioning kidneys were left in place.

Later, I was struck by the magnitude of Erik's role in the surgery compared to Hans'. Erik paved the way, giving up a kidney and jeopardizing his own health and comfort to ensure a healthy, promising life for his brother. Hans followed, receiving the fruit of Erik's surgery.

Afterwards, when friends came by to visit them, Erik was clearly the hero. All thanks, praise and credit went to him. Hans was merely acknowledged as a very fortunate person, and rightly so.

Chapter 2b:
Jesus Paves the Way

In the darkness of Gethsemane, Jesus' disciple Judas betrayed Jesus. Judas led soldiers to Jesus, who surrendered himself without a fight. As soldiers seized him, his friends scattered into the night, leaving Jesus to stand on his own. He was taken to a group of hostile religious leaders who put him on trial. People pounced on him with lies and accusations. Only one held true: Jesus confessed to being the Son of God, thus sealing his own fate.

They charged him with blasphemy, which under Jewish law warranted the death penalty. They took him to Pilate, the governor, because under Roman law they were not allowed to execute a man themselves. Pilate saw no guilt in Jesus, but the religious leaders who opposed Jesus manipulated Pilate by saying Jesus claimed to be the king of the Jews and therefore threatened Caesar's authority. They rallied the crowds who demanded crucifixion. Afraid, Pilate gave Jesus over to Roman soldiers who mocked, whipped and beat him. Then Pilate presented Jesus to the people again, who still insisted on crucifixion. Pilate complied, handing Jesus over for execution.

Jesus was marched through Jerusalem to the outskirts of the city. He was nailed to a cross to pay for his crime like a common criminal, but what he was paying for was the sin of the world. This had been the plan all along.

Jesus' mother Mary, some other devoted women and the disciple John looked on from a distance, unable to help him. Never had Jesus been so alone. On the cross, Jesus took sin upon himself — all of it — past, present and future. The resulting alienation from God's presence was agonizing. Many theologians believe the social, emotional and spiritual anguish of being separated from his Father was more difficult to bear than the awful physical pain.

Just as Erik preceded Hans in the transplant, Jesus preceded us in salvation. Jesus took the initiative without guarantees of cooperation on anyone's part. He laid down his life in a hostile world. To the very end he was mocked and challenged to come down from the cross. His commitment to the cross while people were sinners and enemies of God is incredible. Jesus chose to complete his mission by going through with the "operation" of crucifixion, not for his sake, but ours. This is why Jesus is Savior.

Just like Hans, we are faced with a choice. When you read about Hans' choice to accept Erik's kidney, you might have thought it was a silly point to include. He would have been crazy not to receive the kidney. Erik's offer was practically irresistible. Yet the opportunity to receive the life Jesus offers is even more compelling.

The condition of sin – the universal human "disease" — separates us from God. Sin shows itself through actions and thoughts that hurt others and us, robbing us of right relationship with God and other people. Reconciliation with God begins and ends in what Jesus offered on the cross: his very life. Just as Erik went first and made his kidney available, Jesus went first to reunite us with God.

Jesus laid down his life to usher us into God's presence, now and eternally. He paved the way and made it possible. His part, like Erik's, was big. Our part is to receive Jesus' gift. Our part, like Hans', is small. We simply accept what Jesus offers.

There is therefore no room for human credit in salvation even though we have free will. "For it is by grace you have been saved, through faith — and this not from yourselves, it is the gift of God — not by works, so that no one can boast." (Ephesians 2:8-9)

Just as Erik was the hero in Hans' restoration, Jesus is the hero in our salvation. All the praise, thanks and credit go to him.

The account of Jesus' arrest, trial and crucifixion are found in Matthew 26-27, Mark 14-15, Luke 22-23 and John 18-19. The exclusion of human credit in salvation is discussed in Romans 3-5, Galatians, and Ephesians 2.

But he
was pierced
for our transgressions,
he was crushed for our
iniquities; the punishment that
brought us peace was upon
him, and by his wounds
we are healed.
Isaiah 53:5

Chapter 3a:
Erik's Suffering

Following the surgery Erik had pain in his abdomen, pain from his incisions, and intense pain in his shoulders, neck and upper back. His pain was complicated by the fact that he was not responding to morphine and needed special pain medicine. The pain began Tuesday and continued into Wednesday.

The memory embedded in my mind was the evening Erik's pain medication completely ran out. Erik was in bed crying. His mother was standing at the end of the bed, tears streaming down her face.

She had already informed and then bombarded the nurse's station twice with the request for more pain medication. It took time because the doctor needed to special order it and the pharmacy needed to send it up to our floor.

The situation became more intense as Erik cried harder and nobody could do anything except wait for the medicine to arrive. Mom became increasingly upset, and Tom looked on horrified. Tom, Hans' youngest brother, wanted to be the donor, and now the donor was really suffering. This could have been him! Sarah, who has since become Erik's wife, was sweet and supportive to Erik throughout the ordeal. She sat by his bedside holding his hand. Hans, who was already up and about, looked on feeling helpless.

I stood in the doorway of Erik's room watching the whole scene and feeling detached, as if seeing a movie. Erik's crying had turned to screaming, although he was not angry or yelling. He was experiencing the full weight of his decision as a donor. He knew in advance that the days right after the transplant might be particularly difficult and painful. That's part of why his choice was so significant.

Now he was experiencing that pain. I felt upset that the staff couldn't alleviate his pain more quickly. But even in the midst of such severe pain, I didn't feel an iota of regret that Erik had given his kidney to Hans. I reflected on how his suffering was a direct consequence of my husband's need for a kidney and Erik's willingness to donate it. There was a reason he'd gone through all this: Hans' healing. And so I looked on that evening feeling thankful not only for Erik's choice to donate, but for his tremendous sacrifice as well.

Finally the pain medication came. As it began to work, Erik calmed down and was able to speak again. Sarah was still holding his hand, gazing at him with great concern. Erik looked up at her and encouraged her saying, "Don't worry about me. I'll be okay. I would do it all over again for my brother."

Erik, even in his pain, remembered what the transplant was all about. It was not about suffering, but saving his brother's life. And even after experiencing the pain, he was willing to do it again. Erik's motivation was so pure that even under the duress of pain he did not lash out at Hans or regret having given his kidney.

Chapter 3b:
Jesus' Suffering

Jesus suffered intense physical pain. From the time of his betrayal in the garden, he was subject to abuse and violence. He was beaten with a staff and whipped nearly to death. A crown of thorns was pressed into his scalp. Stakes were driven through his flesh. He hung on a cross and experienced the slow, torturous process of crucifixion.

I imagine Mary wept as Ann had for Erik. Mary could do nothing to ease the physical pain Jesus endured.

Jesus did not revolt or succumb to the taunts of the crowd, "If you really are the Son of God, save yourself!" Instead of saving himself, he stayed on the cross and saved us. Instead of retaliating he said, "Father, forgive them, for they know not what they do."

Jesus didn't want to suffer, but it was something he willingly faced in order to release humanity from sin and death. Just before he submitted his spirit to God, he proclaimed, "It is finished." Some scholars translate it, "It is accomplished." Jesus was referring to the work he did on the cross. He paid for sin, removing the spiritual barrier between people and God. In Jerusalem, at the instant of his death, the temple curtain ripped down the middle, inviting us into God's presence. Jesus was not a victim. Rather, he was a man with a mission.

Have you ever gazed at a picture or sculpture of Jesus hanging on the cross? Some people feel uncomfortable looking at it, while others feel too comfortable and forget its significance. Look again, and focus on the reason Jesus suffered and died. He achieved our eternal security. He endured the cross *for us.*

It was moving to hear Erik tell Sarah, "I would do it again for my brother." Now look into the eyes of Jesus hanging on the cross and hear him say, "Father, forgive them, for they know not what they do." There is no anger or regret in Jesus' voice, only compassion. Even throughout the pain of crucifixion, Jesus did not take revenge or forget his mission.

Jesus' crucifixion and sacrifice are found in Matthew 27, Mark 15, Luke 23, John 19 and Hebrews 10.

Therefore, if
anyone is in Christ,
he is a new creation;
the old is gone, the new has
come! All this is from
God, who reconciled us to
himself through Christ...
2 Corinthians 5:7-8

But the fruit
of the Spirit is
love, joy, peace,
patience, kindness, goodness,
faithfulness, gentleness
and self-control.
Galatians 5:22

Chapter 4a:
Hans' Transformation

Two days after the transplant, life was hectic. It was raining as I dropped off the children at school and got on the Schuylkill Expressway, nicknamed the "Sure Kill" Expressway by some people, because it is narrow, curvy and congested. Normally I avoid this road, but it's a direct route to the hospital, and rush hour was over. Still, the expressway was as crazy as ever. The road was slippery, and I clutched the steering wheel with both hands knowing an accident was the last thing I needed. I was stressed out when I finally exited at South Street.

The hospital was only a few blocks away and soon I entered the parking garage. I groaned since it appeared full. I planned on being at the hospital most of the day so I looked hard for a legitimate space. It took fifteen minutes to find one, and I felt irritated about being charged for this time. Then I negotiated the maze of staircases, walkways, lobbies, hallways and elevators, finally reaching my husband's room.

I wish I could say I collected myself and quietly entered Hans' room, giving him a kiss and my full attention. Instead, I flew into his room and immediately began babbling about the kids starting school, the Schuylkill, the rain, the traffic and the parking. Then I noticed some new flowers and food gifts and began firing questions at him, barely giving him a chance to answer.

Suddenly I noticed something was different. I looked around the room and at Hans. I had come in frazzled, but now I noticed the atmosphere around me was quiet and calm. I stared at Hans. Something struck me as very odd, but what was it? Hans was sitting up in bed, listening to me intently. In his white hospital gown he looked something like an angel, his face glowing. It had color and was peaceful. As I studied him, I realized what was so different: he was sitting *completely still*, able to focus on what I was saying. It was the first time I'd seen him sit still in three months, and the stillest I'd seen him in years.

I forgot my idle chatter and asked, "What is your kidney function this morning? You look wonderful!"

"It's nearly perfect," he grinned. (Two days earlier it was about 9%.) "Erik's kidney is working in me even faster than the doctors predicted. I think my kidney function is higher than Erik's today!"

I was dumbfounded. No wonder he seemed different; he *was* different. Now that Erik's kidney was doing its work in Hans' body by eliminating the toxins, Hans' blood was clean. This allowed him to sit still and relax. The peace produced from within was exuding all around him. Hans was a new man, transformed by Erik's kidney.

I marveled at how Erik was down the hall in his own room. Erik was a whole, functioning human being, yet his kidney was inside Hans making him well.

Chapter 4b:
Our Transformation

Seeing Hans so changed that morning gave new meaning to 2 Corinthians 5:17: "Therefore, if anyone is in Christ, he is a new creation; the old has gone, the new has come." Hans was definitely new and transformed, and I realized that just as Erik models Jesus, Erik's kidney models the Holy Spirit. Jesus can work in us when his Holy Spirit is inside us the same way Erik's kidney works inside Hans. The Holy Spirit purifies our inner being the way Erik's kidney purifies Hans' blood.

Hans didn't get his own kidneys fixed. He got a new kidney — a fresh start. Likewise, we don't get a spiritual band-aid from God, but a whole new deal. When we trust in Jesus and receive his Holy Spirit we are considered new creations. The old life is past and a more excellent life emerges.

When Christians invite others to "accept Jesus," they are talking about receiving and yielding to Jesus' spirit, which is the Holy Spirit. Unlike a kidney though, the Holy Spirit is personal. During his life on earth, Jesus often spoke of the Holy Spirit and promised he would send him to help, guide and transform us. Jesus wants to be with each one of us, and through means of his Holy Spirit, he really can do it. Erik had only one kidney to donate, but Jesus can give the Holy Spirit to *all* who ask him!

When Hans received Erik's kidney, his blood chemistry and demeanor were quickly transformed. Similarly, when someone experiences conversion, he or she may experience some big changes right away. This spiritual change and newness is called being "born again," "born anew," or "born of God." (John 3:3) Many people become aware of specific sins in their life and turn away from them. Many experience peace as they've never known before, others intense joy. Some are miraculously delivered from addictions. Whatever the change, it is not contrived but comes from within.

Receiving the Holy Spirit is the beginning of experiencing life to the fullest. Jesus said, "I came that you may have life, and have it abundantly." (John 10:10) He wants to bring good things into our life. When I saw Hans at peace that morning, it brought to mind the evidence of the Holy Spirit bringing good things into someone's life. It is called the Spirit's "fruit", and includes love, joy, peace, patience, kindness, goodness, faithfulness, gentleness and self-control. (Galatians 5:22)

Viewing the Holy Spirit like a kidney also helps understand the Trinity, which recognizes God's oneness, but in three persons: God the Father, God the Son — Jesus, and God the Holy Spirit. The

Trinity is more traditionally understood through examples like the sun, which is heat, light and mass; or an egg, which is yolk, white and shell; or water, always two parts hydrogen and one part oxygen, but existing in three forms: ice, liquid water and steam. But these examples don't reflect how the Trinity relates to us.

Think of it this way: God is spirit, and Jesus has the very "DNA" of God — the complete divine nature — but in human form. And the Holy Spirit is like a spiritual kidney from Jesus. It is the Spirit of God packaged in a way we can receive in our earthly bodies.

Stop and ponder this mystery a moment: the Spirit of God residing within us. This is not religion, but relationship! It is an awesome thing to experience the love and guidance of God in our lives through the Holy Spirit. He is the ultimate source of confidence and esteem. The Holy Spirit assures us we are children of God and belong to him. His presence within us is something no one can ever snatch away.

Some teachings on the Holy Spirit are found in John 14-16 and Romans 8.

No, in all these things
we are more than conquerors
through him who loved us.
Romans 8:37

Let us fix
our eyes on Jesus,
the author and perfecter of
our faith, who for the joy set
before him endured the cross,
scorning its shame, and
sat down at the right
hand of God.
Hebrews 12:2

Chapter 5a:
Erik's Recovery

Erik endured two days and nights of pain, but on Thursday he was much improved and by Friday he felt ready to leave the hospital. On Saturday, Erik announced he was going whether released or not. The doctors agreed to send both Erik and Hans home.

Hans was happy and peaceful, but his eight-inch incision was tender and he had no intention of walking all the way out of the big hospital. He prudently made use of the wheelchair. Erik, on the other hand, not only walked, but insisted on pushing Hans' wheelchair. It was amazing to see Erik, who just days earlier writhed in pain, taking charge and looking so well.

In fairness to Erik and anyone considering donating a kidney, please know while it is true that Erik wheeled Hans out of the hospital, he did not work for two months. A recovery of four to six weeks is considered standard for a donor whose kidney is removed laparoscopically, but the body's response to surgery varies widely from person to person.

Chapter 5b:
Jesus' Resurrection

In addition to enduring rejection and pain, Jesus experienced death. After Jesus announced he had accomplished what he'd come to do, he said, "Father, into your hands I commit my spirit." Right after this he stopped breathing. Darkness had fallen over the land although it was early afternoon, and at the moment of his death there was an earthquake. A Roman centurion stationed at the cross was so impressed with Jesus, the dignity with which he died, and these powerful events that he proclaimed, "Surely this was the Son of God!"

Before Jesus was removed from the cross, a soldier thrust a spear into Jesus' side to be absolutely sure he was dead. Immediately water and blood gushed out, indicating Jesus' heart had been pierced.*

Despite Jesus' alleged crimes, Pilate allowed Jesus a proper burial. Joseph and Nicodemus, religious leaders who revered Jesus, placed his dead body in a tomb. A large boulder was rolled in front of the tomb, and Roman soldiers were sent to guard it. But a tomb could not hold him. On the third day, Jesus rose from the dead just as he had told his disciples he would. For the next forty days Jesus appeared to hundreds, showing them he was alive, teaching from the Scriptures, and promising to send his Holy Spirit once he returned to the Father.

The resurrection asserts the truth of Jesus' claims, predictions and promises. It assures us of the effective work of the crucifixion. Though Jesus' human body died, sacrificed for our sin, he rose in power with a resurrected, heavenly body. We serve and honor a *living* Jesus. He has overcome sin and death. He is victor, king and Lord.

Dying for our sins was not the end of the story. The passion of Jesus is not one of punishment, death, decay and despair; rather it is about choice, sacrifice, love and triumph.

*NIV text note John 19:34

Jesus' death and resurrection are found in Matthew 27-28, Mark 15-16, Luke 23-24 and John 19-20.

Do not be conformed
any longer to the pattern of this
world, but be transformed by
the renewing of your mind.
Romans 12:2

….being confident
of this, that he who began
a good work in you will carry
it on to completion…
Philippians 1:6

Chapter 6a:
Adjusting to the Kidney

Remember how Hans looked like an angel, peaceful and still because of Erik's kidney? I wish it was the end of the story, but instead it was a new beginning. Hans had a bright future but also had some struggles ahead of him.

When Hans left the hospital the doctors prescribed all sorts of medications — antibacterial, antiviral and anti-rejection — a regimen of nearly 40 pills a day that would taper down over the months ahead. These medications would keep his immune system from attacking and rejecting the kidney, which Hans' body viewed as an alien invader. Even though Erik's kidney was a perfect match, Hans' body was hostile toward the kidney and needed time to adjust to it being there. Because the medications suppress the immune system, Hans was told to avoid germs since he was especially vulnerable to contracting illnesses during this time.

With young children in the house, the first six months were difficult. Our youngest son caught Fifth Disease and spread it to Hans. (Fifth Disease produces the "fifth" childhood rash and is caused by a virus.) Hans experienced extreme fatigue and low hemoglobin, ending up in the hospital for several days. It wasn't even Christmas and I wondered how Hans would make it through the winter with colds and the flu going around. But he did, and by spring Hans was healthy and taking fewer medications, down to ten pills a day.

Now, years later, Hans no longer needs to worry about avoiding germs. Erik's kidney is working well and has made its home in Hans. He looks completely healthy and is very active. When I tell people he had a kidney transplant when he was 35, they are surprised because no one would guess he had ever been so sick.

Hans is grateful to be alive and able to travel. Because he is healthy and not tied to dialysis, he has the stamina and freedom to hike mountains and take long trips. After the transplant, Hans climbed Mt. Washington in New Hampshire and took a month long vacation to explore the West. This level of activity and geographical range would not be possible without Erik's kidney.

Hans realizes this and takes care of the kidney. He nurtures the gift Erik has given him by taking his medications, drinking plenty of water, eating healthy, exercising, sleeping and visiting the doctor several times a year. He doesn't do these things out of obligation to Erik, but for his own good, because he values the kidney.

Chapter 6b:
Living with the Spirit

When the Holy Spirit first comes and dwells in us some wonderful changes may take place, but it isn't the end. Instead, it's the beginning of a whole new life, one of walking with God. It's like when Hans was transformed overnight, which was exciting and amazing, but then his body requires a lifetime of commitment and care. It's the same with spiritual birth; something new and wonderful has come, but there is a challenging road ahead.

The problem is, just as Hans' body initially attacked Erik's kidney, our body wages war against the Holy

Spirit. There is a power struggle going on within us: our sinful nature is in conflict with God's nature. Our desires don't always line up with God's will, and the Holy Spirit living within us wants *his* way with us. We need to grow in harmony with the Holy Spirit just as Hans' body adjusted to the new kidney.

Just as Hans tried to avoid germs for a while, we benefit from initially avoiding tempting situations and bad influences. And just as Hans contracted Fifth Disease, we should not become discouraged when we initially experience failures and setbacks walking with God. As time goes by, we become better able to follow the guidance of the Spirit. The Spirit changes us from within, and our flesh is no longer fighting against the Spirit but is in sync with it. More and more we embrace the things of God, and slowly but surely God's desires become our desires. This is a process of coming into agreement with God.

As a result, we become more resilient spiritually and are better able to face temptation, just as over that first year Hans became more able to combat germs. We move from a defensive position, which involves getting free from sin, to an offensive position, which involves furthering the kingdom of God. Our body stops fighting the Holy Spirit and makes peace so they begin working together. Now God can literally work through us because his Holy Spirit is in us, and we are in step with him rather than struggling against him. Consequently we become "God's hands and feet," — his instruments of service on the earth.

A word of caution: we must never get too comfortable and forget the Spirit, or become arrogant and take over. We need to continually rely on the Holy Spirit's strength and direction. The Apostle Paul once scolded some Christians, "Are you so foolish? After beginning with the Spirit, are you now trying to attain your goal by human effort?" (Galatians 3:3)

It is human nature to want control and predictability, turning to rules, laws, lists and formulas. It is the kidney that began the miracle in Hans, and it is the kidney that will continue to keep him well. Likewise, it is the Holy Spirit who transforms us spiritually, and it is the Holy Spirit who will keep us on track.

Getting a kidney meant freedom for Hans, not to foolishly ignore his health, but to reach his potential and go places. Receiving the Holy Spirit also brings freedom, not to sin, but to reach our potential in God, which is our full potential as human beings. We experience freedom from sin and guilt, freedom from striving, and freedom from sacrifices and lists of rules. "Now the Lord is the Spirit, and where the Spirit of the Lord is there is freedom." (2 Corinthians 3:17)

Just as Hans has ways of caring for his kidney, there are ways to foster the Holy Spirit in our life. Here are a few:

Prayer — talking with God, listening to God;

Fellowship — meeting with other people who encourage us in our faith;

Worship — submitting our will and plans to God; loving God and other people;

Praise — giving God honor and thanks through word or song;

Bible study — reading or listening to the Bible, meditating on it and then applying it;

These are a few of the disciplines that provide the Holy Spirit within us a positive, pure environment for a healthy start and solid future. As we continue to grow spiritually, we devote ourselves to these spiritual disciplines not out of religious duty to God, but because they are good for us and we treasure the gift of the Holy Spirit.

The struggle between the Holy Spirit and our human desires is found in Romans 7-8 and Galatians 5.

We know that we
live in him and he in us,
because he has given
us of his Spirit.
1 John 4:13

The Spirit himself
testifies with our spirit
that we are God's children.
Romans 8:16

…this mystery
which is Christ in you,
the hope of glory.
Colossians 1:27

Chapter 7a:
Becoming Like Erik

I had always viewed Erik and Hans as being cut from different molds. Although both men are smart, creative and entrepreneurial, their appearance and personalities are quite different. Erik is tall and slim, while Hans is solid with broad shoulders. Erik is sweet, charming and intuitive. Hans is serious, more reserved and analytical. On that basis I had falsely reasoned that Erik becoming the donor was unrealistic. But something curious happened after the kidney transplant: Hans started eating, looking and behaving more like Erik.

The first thing we noticed was Hans' appetite. For the first time in our married life Hans was hungry for seconds at dinner. We think his hunger was a response to one of the medicines he was taking, but it reminded me so much of Erik's big appetite.

The second thing that changed was his beverage preference. Prior to the transplant, Hans drank about a gallon of water and three or four soft drinks a day. After the transplant he continued to drink lots of water but couldn't stand the taste of soda. A few times he poured a soda but would not finish it because it tasted awful.

Instead, Hans began to enjoy coffee. Whereas he had very little interest in coffee before the transplant, for the first time Starbucks appeared on our credit card statement. One day Hans phoned Erik on an inkling and asked him what he drinks. It turns out Erik doesn't drink much soda but loves coffee!

Our friend Elizabeth pointed out a third change: "Hans is so different now; he was talking to me the other day and he was animated and downright social." We discussed that this was probably the result of Hans being healthy and energetic for the first time in years, but I had one other idea. "Erik's friendly and nice to talk with. You know, Erik's DNA is all over the kidney inside Hans, and it's filtering all his blood. Hey, maybe Erik's charm will rub off on Hans too!"

I am still adjusting to a fourth, highly visual change. Before the transplant, Hans' hair was straight. Within a year of the surgery, Hans' hair looked curly just like Erik's. I have known Hans since junior high and his hair has always been blond and straight. Now his hair is darker and can get pretty curly and wild looking, especially on humid days. At first it startled me: "Who are you and what have you done with my husband?" We assume his sudden hair change is a result of the medications, but when Hans and Erik are together, their hair is so much alike we wonder if there isn't more to it.

I thought Hans and Erik were very different, but now they really seem a lot alike. We understand the changes Hans experienced are probably responses to medications and improved health, but we joke that kidneys do all kinds of things medical science has yet to uncover!

Chapter 7b:
Becoming Like Jesus

I t has been fun to see Hans looking and acting more like Erik because it presents this parallel: when the Holy Spirit resides in us, we start looking and acting more like Jesus. We become like Jesus not only because we follow his teachings, but also because he is living inside us through his Holy Spirit. He is changing us into his likeness from within!

The Holy Spirit makes us hungry like Hans, not for food, but for spiritual things. Before receiving the Holy Spirit, we may have dreaded church and the people there. The Bible seemed boring or incomprehensible, prayer felt foolish, and there was no desire to worship God. But with the Holy Spirit living inside us, this changes. A spiritual appetite develops for his word, his will, his work and his church.

While the desire for godly things increases, the taste for harmful or evil things decreases. As Hans lost his taste for soda, we might lose our taste for certain television shows, activities or patterns of behavior. Our preferences and priorities morph over time through a process called sanctification, in which God touches all the areas of our life and makes them holy and good. It's not that he doesn't love us the way we are, but for our own sake he doesn't leave areas of sin in our life anymore than we would leave a baby in a dirty diaper.

The Holy Spirit also affects the way we interact with people. Just as Hans became more outgoing, the Holy Spirit helps us get along with others better. The Holy Spirit produces love, joy, peace, patience, kindness, goodness, faithfulness, gentleness and self-control. Concurrently, the Holy Spirit does away with anger, jealousy, hatred, pride and selfish ambition. (Galatians 5:20-23)

For example, if we are in the habit of angrily yelling at family members, the Holy Spirit will help us be patient and loving to them instead. If we are in the habit of gossiping, the Holy Spirit will help us use our tongue to encourage others. It is no wonder that our relationships will improve!

Last, the Holy Spirit will make us look different. It might not be as obvious as Hans' curly hair, but it will show. Maybe our face will shine with joy instead of sorrow, or peace instead of anxiety. Maybe our stride will become more humble. Maybe our likeness to Jesus will become apparent as we serve or extend hospitality. Maybe we never cared about other people, and now we do. Whatever the change, we will look more like Jesus than when his Spirit first came into our life.

If you then,
though you are evil,
know how to give good gifts
to your children, how much
more will your Father in
heaven give the Holy Spirit to
those who ask him!
Luke 11:13

And hope
does not disappoint us,
because God has poured out
his love into our hearts by the
Holy Spirit whom he
has given us.
Romans 5:5

Chapter 8a:
Perfect Match

Hans had three options when he was sick. One option was to do nothing. He could have disregarded his declining health and died prematurely.

His second option was dialysis. He could go to a dialysis unit three times a week and have his blood filtered by a machine. He would have clean blood when he left the unit, but over a couple days, toxins and fluids building up in his bloodstream would create the need for another filtering. This regimen would require monitoring fluid intake and keeping travel away from the dialysis unit to three days.

Dialysis could keep him alive but would need to be repeated over and over. It is seen as a means to sustain life until a transplant can be arranged and is not considered a permanent solution by doctors or the insurance industry. Many people are kept alive by dialysis but it wears hard on the body. Therefore, in most cases dialysis is viewed as a waiting place or holding pattern.

Hans' third option was to have a transplant and receive a perfectly matched kidney. Choosing this option would include saying yes to Erik's offer, surgery with general anesthesia, an eight-inch incision, several months of recovery and medications for life. The transplant would allow Hans to be independent. He would be healthy and could travel anywhere for any length of time.

The choice was obvious for Hans. The perfectly matched kidney offered health and freedom.

Hans was fortunate to have four brothers willing to consider donation. He was very fortunate to have the option of a perfect match. To get a perfect match from a stranger is extremely rare. If someone dies in the United States and his kidney is cleared for donation, his blood type and six antigens are checked against a national transplant waiting list. If the blood type and six antigens all match, the kidney will be flown to the transplant patient's location, even if it's clear across the country. Getting a perfect match from a stranger is like winning the lottery.

Most people do not get a perfect match. They get a good match, in which the blood type is compatible and one or more of the six antigens match. Even so, many people wait a long, long time. Some people die waiting.

Chapter 8b:
Perfect Match

On a spiritual level, we have the same three options Hans had. One is to do nothing about sin, the universal "disease." When one of Hans' options was to do nothing about his illness, did it sound ridiculous? Yet it would be even more negligent to ignore the condition of sin.

We desire to be loved and known for who we truly are, but only God knows us completely and loves us unconditionally. Yet we look for fulfillment in other people, the pursuit of power or position, and material possessions. This waywardness of ours that wanders and seeks independence from God is called sin. Many people think sin is just about doing horrible things like murder, but the root of sin is rebellion, however subtle or overt. Since God is our creator he knows what's best for us and we fall under his authority, but we often ignore or forget him and run our own life.

Many of the effects of sin are inside and hidden, just like the long-term effects of Hans' kidney illness. Hans didn't look or feel sick when he was diagnosed as a teenager. Even years later when he needed a transplant he didn't understand just how very sick he was, because over the years he adjusted to his illness. A year *after* the transplant Hans commented, "I can play sports better. There's freedom in my joints and I'm more limber. Now that I'm well, I understand how much my kidney illness affected my entire body."

Then Hans made this parallel: "Humans live in a condition of sin. We're used to it and we accept it as if it's normal. But when the Holy Spirit does his work in us and we experience God's presence, then we understand how much sin affected us before."

Therefore, it's easy to ignore sin, and it's important to come to terms with sin lest we miss out on all that God has for us.

The second option for addressing sin is "religious dialysis." In this case, there is no denial about sin, but there is the notion we can overcome it the self-help way. This involves offering sacrifices, doing service or behaving morally in order to compensate for sin, and then repeating the actions over and over again. It never completely clears the conscience or puts us in right relationship with God.

"Religious dialysis" could be anything that involves trying to achieve salvation without the Savior. The idea of earning our own salvation is futile, exhausting, and doesn't address the root problem. The Bible makes it clear, beginning with Abraham, that we are saved by faith in God who can save us, not by our own works and devising. Scripture also reveals that the sacrificial system pointed to, led to, and ended with Jesus' complete and perfect sacrifice on the cross.

The third option for addressing sin is to get a transplant, in which the living God comes to renew us through his Holy Spirit. This is God's solution, and his desire for us all. This is the option that promises abundant and eternal life, peace with God, and freedom from guilt and sin.

Why then is there ever resistance? Sometimes the same sin that needs healing rears its ugly head in the form of pride. We take pride in our autonomy. Independence is highly valued in our culture. Some people feel receiving help from God exhibits weakness and is a crutch. Salvation is a gift we don't deserve, and we struggle with receiving something for which we haven't worked and can't reciprocate.

So then, how do we receive the gift of salvation, not by merit or work, but in faith and humility? Hans' situation provides a clue. He received Erik's kidney because he understood enough about his illness to want the promising life the kidney offered. Similarly, we receive Jesus' gift of salvation when we grasp our spiritual illness. Do we understand our sinful condition and how it hurts us? Can we put aside our pride and say yes to all God offers us? If yes, we are ready for a spiritual transplant.

Since Jesus came to earth as a human being, made like us in every way, he is a Perfect Match. He is a 100% compatible donor. Since he initiated the process through his death on the cross, the hard part is already done. Relationship with God through the Holy Spirit is available today. There is no waiting list!

The months preceding the transplant, Hans knew Erik was a perfect match and understood how a transplant worked. Yet he could be sitting right next to Erik and still be sick. In order for Hans to actually be healed, he needed to have surgery and the kidney placed inside him.

Jesus is a perfect match for us, able to cure our sin. We may know about Jesus and understand Biblical truths intellectually. We may even attend church each week but still be spiritually broken because head knowledge is not the key.

Remember the disciples arguing at the last Passover, sleeping in Gethsemane when Jesus asked for support, and fleeing when Jesus was arrested? Even though these men had been Jesus' constant companions for three years, they needed Jesus' Spirit inside of them to really change. After his ascension, Jesus sent his disciples the Holy Spirit. They went from being cowards to boldly spreading the news of Jesus and doing miracles in his name.

Likewise, in order for us to be truly changed, we too need Jesus' Spirit. Begin by making an appointment with Jesus, the Great Physician. Get on the "operating table" and open your life to him. Ask for his Spirit with confidence, because he is a Perfect Match! Jesus will not deny you for he said, "Ask, and it will be given you. For everyone who asks receives. If you then, though you are evil, know how to give good gifts to your children, how much more will your Father in heaven give the Holy Spirit to those who ask him!" (Luke 11:9,10,13)

For God did not send
his Son into the world to
condemn the world, but to
save the world through him.
John 3:17

Jesus stood and said
in a loud voice, "If anyone
is thirsty, let him come to me
and drink. Whoever believes
in me, as the Scripture has
said, streams of living water
will flow from within him."
By this he meant the Spirit,
whom those who believed in
him were later to receive. Up
to that time the Spirit had not
been given, since Jesus had
not yet been glorified.
John 7:37-39

Endnote

Although each chapter in *Perfect Match* presents its own point, there are two main streams of thought throughout the book.

First, Jesus is not simply a good teacher or prophet from the past. He is the Son of God, and no one compares to him. He is Savior and Lord. Jesus is alive and seeks relationship with us through his Holy Spirit. He is not the son of a vengeful or distant God. Rather, Jesus demonstrates the love of God.

Second, the Holy Spirit is the key to spirituality because the Holy Spirit *is* the *Spirit* of God. The Holy Spirit can heal and transform a life once he comes in.

We can nurture the gift of the Holy Spirit through disciplines like prayer, Bible study and worship. If you are not involved already, I urge you to seek out a church, fellowship, Alpha course or Bible study where you will be encouraged to grow in your faith.

My husband was restored physically. Regrettably, many patients aren't that fortunate since there is a shortage of available kidneys. **But everyone can receive the perfect match Jesus offers: the Holy Spirit, who brings abundant, eternal life.**

Hopefully Erik's kidney will see Hans through this life; we are not sure how long it will last. But the perfect match Jesus offers, the Holy Spirit, promises to take us through this life and into eternity. What Jesus offers is a sure thing — there is no shortage of his Holy Spirit or his love.

If you desire to get a "spiritual transplant," you may anywhere, anytime. You begin by simply talking to God. The prayer below can help you get started. Then continue as the Spirit leads. Always take time to listen when you pray.

God, thank you that through your son Jesus you came to earth and died for our sins. Please forgive me for the things I do wrong and for going my own direction. Please come into my life through your Holy Spirit. Please purify me, transform me and guide me. Please help and strengthen me to do your will always.

To purchase additional copies:

www.amazon.com

Printed in the United States
54793LVS00001B/253-333

9 781600 341434